DINNER&SNACK

n. 25 Recipes for Dinner &
n.25 Types of Snack
28-DAY MEAL PLAN

HELENA DIAS SCOTT

Table of Contents

DINNER RECIPES

1. Chicken Breast and Bok Choy in Parchment

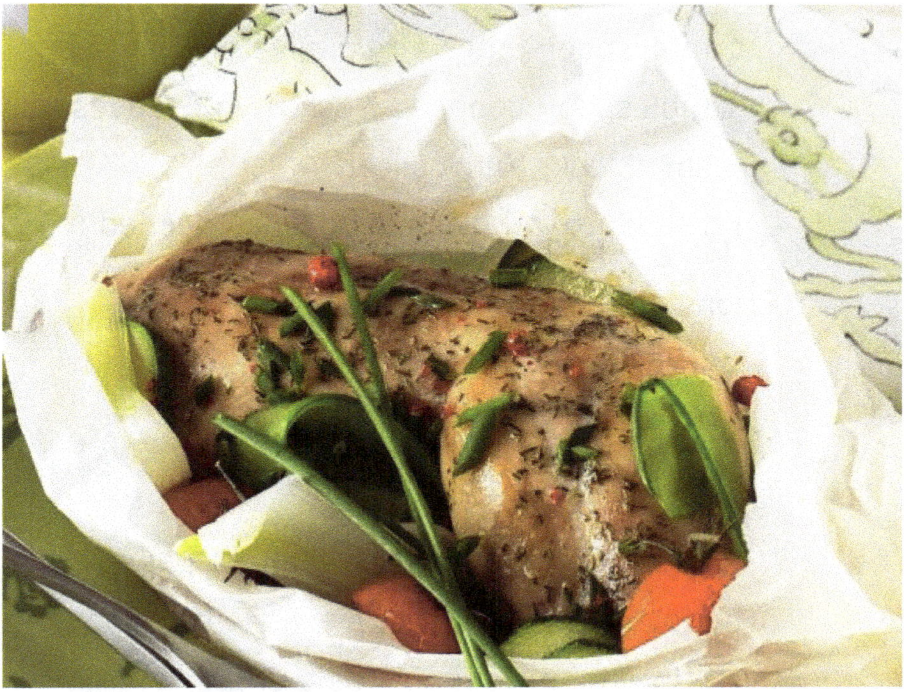

Preparation Time: 10 minutes

Cooking time: 30 minutes

Servings: 4

Ingredients:

- 4 boneless, skinless chicken breasts

- 4 lemon slices
- 2 carrots, julienned
- 2 cups thinly sliced Bok choy
- 1 tablespoon Dijon mustard
- 1 tablespoon extra-virgin olive oil
- 1 tablespoon chopped fresh thyme leaves
- 1 small leek, thinly sliced
- Freshly ground black pepper, as needed

Directions:

1. Preheat the oven to 425 F.
2. Mix the mustard, olive oil, and thyme in your small bowl.
3. Prepare four pieces of parchment paper by folding four 18-inch pieces in half and cutting them like you would create a heart. Open each piece and lay flat.
4. In each piece of parchment, arrange ½ cup of Bok choy, a small handful of carrots, and a few slices of leek. Place the chicken breast on top, and season with pepper.

5. Brush the marinade over the chicken breasts, and top each with a slice of lemon. Fold the packets shut, and fold the paper along the edges to crease and seal the packages.
6. Cook for 20 minutes. Let rest for 5 minutes, and open carefully to serve.

Nutritional Values: Calories: 164; Total Fat: 5g; Carbohydrates: 8g; Protein: 24g; Fiber: 2g; Phosphorus: 26mg; Potassium: 187mg; Sodium: 356mg; Cholesterol: 72mg; Iron 2.7mg; Vitamin A: 439.8mcg; Vitamin C: 100.5mg

2. Roasted Cod with Plums

Preparation Time: 10 minutes

Cooking time: 20 minutes

Servings: 4

Ingredients:

- 6 red plums, halved and pitted

- 1½ pounds cod fillets
- 3 tablespoons extra-virgin olive oil
- 2 tablespoons freshly squeezed lemon juice
- ½ teaspoon dried thyme leaves
- 1/8 teaspoon salt
- 1/8 teaspoon freshly ground black pepper
- ¾ cup plain whole-milk yogurt, for serving

Directions:

1. Warm your oven to 375 F. Line a baking sheet using parchment paper.
2. Arrange the plums, cut-side up, along with the fish on the prepared baking sheet. Drizzle with olive oil and lemon juice and sprinkle with thyme, salt, and pepper.
3. Roast for 15 to 20 minutes or until the fish flakes when tested with a fork and the plums are tender. Serve with yogurt.

Nutritional Values: Calories: 230; Total Fat: 9g; Carbohydrates: 10g; Protein: 27g; Fiber: 1g; Phosphorus: 197mg; Potassium: 437mg; Sodium: 154mg; Cholesterol: 54mg; Iron 4mg; Vitamin A: 503.1mcg; Vitamin C: 32mg

3. Cauliflower and Potato Curry

Preparation Time: 10 minutes

Cooking time: 15 minutes

Servings: 4

Ingredients:

- 2 small tomatoes, diced
- 1 small head cauliflower, cut into florets
- 1 medium potato, diced
- 1 small green chile, stemmed, seeded, and diced
- ½ sweet onion, chopped
- ½ cup water
- ¼ cup chopped cilantro leaves
- 3 garlic cloves, minced

- 2-inch piece ginger
- 2 tablespoons canola oil
- 1 teaspoon ground turmeric
- 1 teaspoon ground cumin
- 1 teaspoon garam masala
- Juice of ½ lemon
- Rice or bread, for serving

Directions:

1. In your large pot over medium heat, heat the olive oil. Add the onion and cook, stirring, until softened.
2. Add the ginger and garlic, and cook until fragrant. Stir in the turmeric and cumin. Add the cauliflower, potato, tomatoes, Chile, and water.
3. Bring to a simmer, reduce the heat, and cover. Cook, occasionally stirring, for 25 minutes, until the potatoes and cauliflower are tender.

4. Stir in the lemon juice, cilantro, and garam masala. Serve over rice or with bread.

Nutritional Values: Calories: 146; Total Fat: 7g; Carbohydrates: 19g; Protein: 3g; Fiber: 3g; Phosphorus: 65mg; Potassium: 546mg; Sodium: 20mg; Cholesterol: 0mg; Iron 2.3mg; Vitamin A: 76.7mcg; Vitamin C: 30mg

4. Flank Steak with Chimichurri Sauce

Preparation Time: 10 minutes

Cooking time: 15 minutes

Servings: 6

Ingredients:

For the chimichurri sauce:

- ¼ cup finely chopped fresh parsley
- ¼ cup finely chopped fresh cilantro
- ¼ cup finely chopped sweet onion
- 2 garlic cloves, minced
- ¼ cup extra-virgin olive oil

- 2 tablespoons apple cider vinegar
- ¼ teaspoon freshly ground black pepper
- ¼ teaspoon red chili flakes

For the steak:

- 1½ pounds flank steak
- 1 teaspoon garlic powder
- ½ teaspoon dried oregano
- Freshly ground black pepper, as needed

Directions:

1. Mix the parsley, cilantro, onion, garlic, olive oil, vinegar, pepper, and chili flakes in a bowl. Keep aside.
2. Preheat the broiler on high. Adjust an oven shelf to be as close to the broiler as possible. Flavor the flank steak on all sides with garlic powder, oregano, and pepper.
3. Place the steak on a wire rack over a baking sheet, and cook for 5 minutes on one side. Flip and cook the other side for

an additional 3 to 5 minutes until the desired doneness.

4. Remove from the oven, and tent the steak with a piece of aluminum foil. Let it rest for 5 minutes. Slice crosswise against the grain, and serve with the chimichurri sauce.

Nutritional Values: Calories: 273; Total Fat: 18g; Carbohydrates: 2g; Protein: 24g; Fiber: 0g; Phosphorus: 226mg; Potassium: 416mg; Sodium: 64mg; Cholesterol: 47.6mg; Iron 4.1mg; Vitamin A: 888.9mcg; Vitamin C: 18mg

5. Peanut-Chili Tofu with Noodles

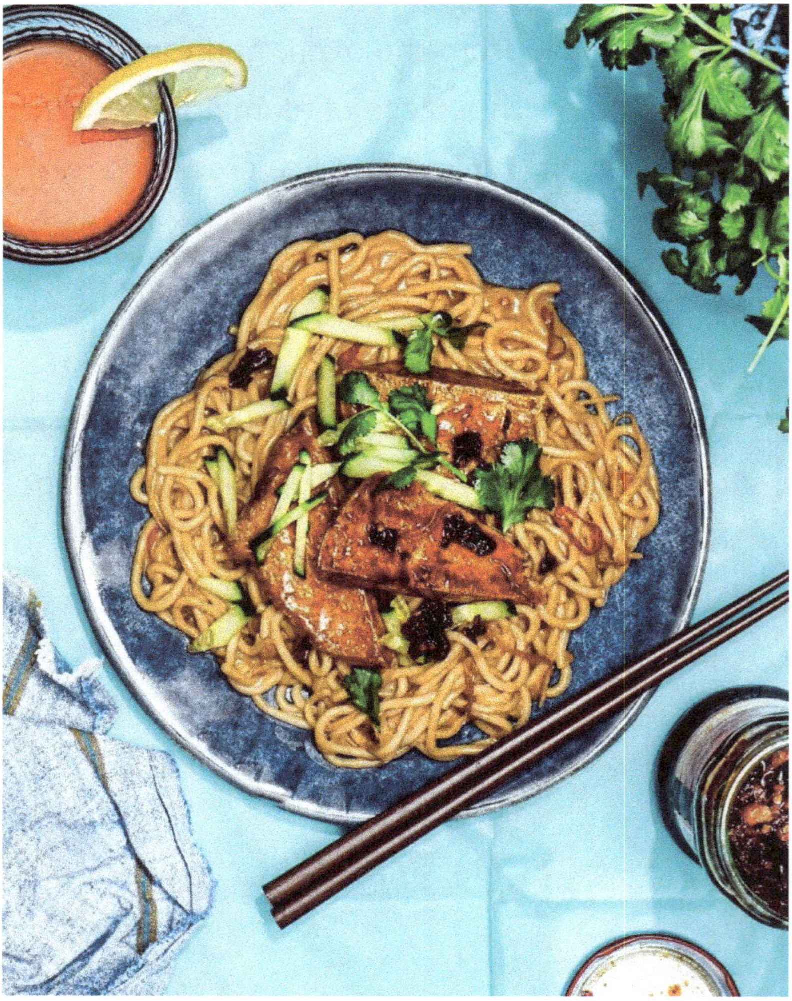

Preparation Time: 10 minutes

Cooking time: 20 minutes

Servings: 2

Ingredients:

- 6 ounces firm tofu, cut into cubes
- 4 ounces dry spaghetti
- 2 garlic cloves, minced
- 1 medium green bell pepper, sliced
- 1 small red onion, chopped
- 1 cup grated carrots
- 2 tablespoons unsalted peanut butter
- 1 tablespoon sesame oil
- 1 tablespoon rice vinegar
- 1 tablespoon minced fresh ginger
- 1 tablespoon olive oil

Directions:

1. Cook the spaghetti as stated in the package directions. Drain and set aside.
2. Mix the peanut butter, sesame oil, rice vinegar, garlic, and ginger in your small bowl. Set aside.

3. In a medium pan over medium heat, heat the olive oil. Add the onion, bell pepper, and carrots and cook until soft, about 5 minutes.
4. Add the tofu to your pan with the vegetables and cook until soft, about 5 minutes.
5. Coat the tofu and vegetables with an 1/8 cup of peanut butter sauce in the same pan.
6. Add the spaghetti noodles and the remaining 1/8 cup of sauce to the tofu and vegetables. Coat and mix everything well.

Nutritional Values: Calories: 557; Protein: 20g; Total Fat: 26g; Carbohydrates: 62g; Fiber: 6.5g; Phosphorus: 208mg; Potassium: 571mg; Sodium: 163mg; Cholesterol: 0mg; Iron 2.4mg; Vitamin A: 133.5mcg; Vitamin C: 23.8mg

6. Lemon Chicken

Preparation Time: 20 minutes

Cooking time: 24 minutes

Servings: 4

Ingredients:

- 12 ounces boneless skinless chicken breasts, cubed
- 2 lemons
- 1 cup 2-inch green bean pieces
- 1 cup 2-inch asparagus pieces
- ½ large onion, chopped
- 2 tablespoons extra-virgin olive oil
- 1/8 teaspoon salt
- 1/8 teaspoon freshly ground black pepper

Directions:

1. Zest 1 of the lemons and pour the zest into a medium bowl. Juice that lemon and add the juice to the bowl. Slice the

remaining lemon, remove the seeds, and set aside.

2. In the bowl with the lemon juice, place the cubed chicken and set aside for 10 minutes to marinate.
3. Heat the olive oil in your large skillet over medium heat.
4. Using a slotted spoon, remove the chicken from the lemon juice, reserving the lemon juice mixture.
5. Add the chicken to the pan and cook for 3 to 4 minutes, stirring, until the chicken is lightly browned. Transfer the chicken to your clean plate and sprinkle with salt and pepper.
6. Add the sliced lemon to the skillet and cook for 3 minutes on each side, turning once, until it is slightly caramelized. Transfer to the plate with the chicken.
7. Add the onion to your skillet and cook within 3 to 4 minutes, until the onion is

tender-crisp, stirring to loosen the chicken drippings from the skillet.

8. Add the green beans and sauté for 2 minutes. Add the asparagus and sauté for 1 minute.
9. Return the chicken to the skillet and add the reserved lemon juice. Simmer for 4 to 6 minutes until the vegetables are tender and the sauce has slightly thickened.
10. Add the caramelized lemon slices to the skillet and cook for 1 to 2 minutes, stirring, until hot. Serve.

Nutritional Values: Calories: 207; Total Fat: 9g; Carbohydrates: 11g; Protein: 22g; Fiber: 4g; Phosphorus: 245mg; Potassium: 593mg; Sodium: 121mg; Cholesterol: 73mg; Iron 0.5mg; Vitamin A: 13mcg; Vitamin C: 8mg

7. Creamy Veggie Casserole

Preparation Time: 25 minutes

Cooking time: 35 minutes

Servings: 4

Ingredients:

- 3 cups frozen California blend vegetables
- 3 cups low-sodium vegetable broth
- 1 cup crushed crisp rice cereal
- 1/3 cup extra-virgin olive oil, divided
- 1 onion, chopped
- 2 tablespoons flour

Directions:

1. Preheat the oven to 375 F.
2. Heat 2 tablespoons of olive oil in your large saucepan over medium heat. Add the onion and cook for 3 to 4 minutes, stirring, until the onion is tender. Add the flour and stir for 2 minutes.
3. Add the broth to the saucepan, stirring for 3 to 4 minutes, or until the sauce thickens.

4. Add the vegetables to the saucepan. Let it simmer and cook within 6 to 8 minutes, or until the vegetables are hot and tender.
5. Pour the mixture into a 3-quart casserole dish when the vegetables are done. Sprinkle the vegetables with the crushed cereal.
6. Bake within 20 to 25 minutes or until the cereal is golden brown and the filling is bubbling. Let cool for 5 minutes and serve.

Nutritional Values: Calories: 234; Total Fat: 18g; Carbohydrates: 16g; Protein: 3g; Fiber: 3g; Phosphorus: 21mg; Potassium: 210mg; Sodium: 139mg; Cholesterol: 50.63mg; Iron 1.32mg; Vitamin A: 876.2mcg; Vitamin C: 28.01mg

8. Salmon and Kale in Parchment

Preparation Time: 10 minutes

Cooking time: 15 minutes

Servings: 4

Ingredients:

- 1 pound salmon fillets
- 4 fresh rosemary sprigs
- 4 fresh thyme sprigs
- 2 cups thinly sliced kale leaves
- 2 small zucchinis, sliced
- 1 lemon, sliced
- ¼ cup dry white wine
- ½ teaspoon paprika
- Freshly ground black pepper, as needed

Directions:

1. Warm your oven to 450 F. Cut four pieces of parchment paper, each about 12 inches in diameter.
2. On each paper lay ½ cup of kale leaves, and top it with several slices of zucchini—season with pepper.

3. Season the salmon fillets with paprika, then top each fillet with a thyme sprig, a rosemary sprig, and a slice of lemon. Pour 1 tablespoon of white wine over each fillet.
4. Fold the parchment paper to join the seams, and crease to form a seal.
5. Bake for 15 minutes. Remove from the oven and let the fillets cool for about 5 minutes before serving.

Nutritional Values: Calories: 201; Total Fat: 7g; Carbohydrates: 60g; Protein: 26g; Fiber: 2g; Phosphorus: 332mg; Potassium: 614mg; Sodium: 144mg; Cholesterol: 85mg; Iron 3mg; Vitamin A: 107.8mcg; Vitamin C: 25.1mg

9. Turkey Meatballs and Spaghetti in

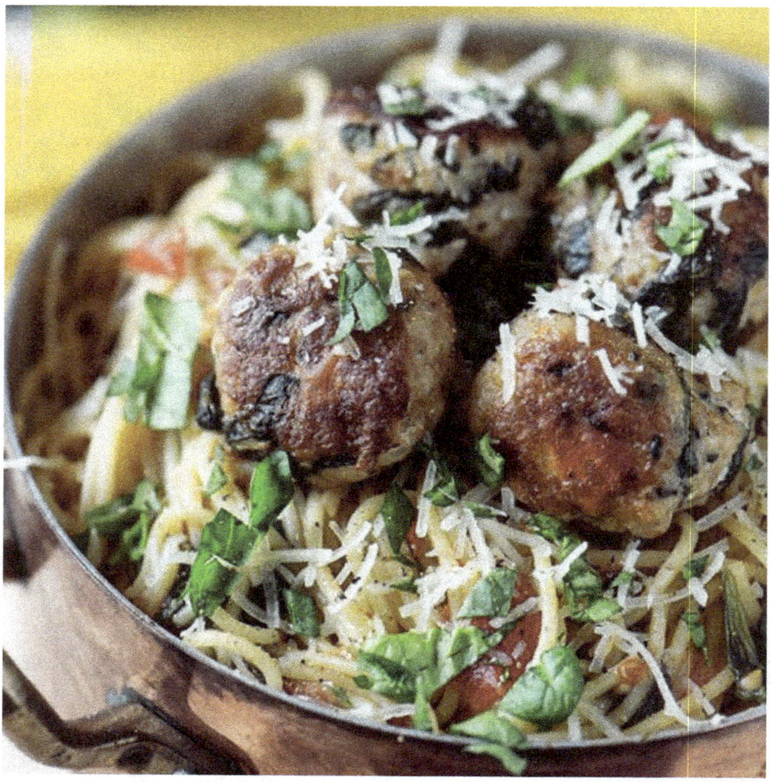

Garlic Sauce

Preparation Time: 15 minutes

Cooking time: 20 minutes

Servings: 4

Ingredients:

For the meatballs:

- ¾ pound lean ground turkey
- 1 large egg, beaten
- ½ cup bread crumbs
- ½ teaspoon onion powder
- ½ teaspoon garlic powder

For the pasta:

- 8 ounces spaghetti noodles
- 5 garlic cloves, minced
- 2 cups chopped broccoli rabe
- ¼ cup shredded Parmesan cheese
- 1 tablespoon extra-virgin olive oil
- Freshly ground black pepper, as needed

Directions:

1. Warm your oven to 375 F. Line a baking sheet with parchment paper.
2. Combine the turkey, bread crumbs, egg, onion powder, and garlic powder in your medium bowl. Mix well.

3. Shape the turkey mixture into 2-inch round meatballs, and place them on the baking sheet.
4. Bake for 20 minutes, until browned and cooked through, flipping the meatballs once halfway through cooking.
5. Let your pot filled with water comes to a boil, and cook the noodles al dente. Drain, reserving about 1 cup of the cooking water.
6. In a large skillet, heat the oil over medium-high heat. Add the garlic and cook until fragrant. Add the broccoli rabe and ½ cup of reserved cooking water to the skillet.
7. Adjust its heat to simmer, cover, and cook for 5 minutes until the broccoli rabe is fork-tender.
8. Add the noodles to the skillet and mix. Add a couple of tablespoons or more of the remaining cooking water to the skillet to wet the noodles.

9. Stir in the Parmesan cheese and season with pepper. Serve the noodles topped with the meatballs.

Nutritional Values: Calories: 450; Total Fat: 15g; Carbohydrates: 55g; Protein: 23g; Fiber: 3g; Phosphorus: 319mg; Potassium: 354mg; Sodium: 245mg; Cholesterol: 105.22mg; Iron 1.9mg; Vitamin A: 0mcg; Vitamin C: 16.1mg

10. Rice-Stuffed Mini Meatloaves

Preparation Time: 20 minutes

Cooking time: 50 minutes

Servings: 5

Ingredients:

- 1¼ pounds extra-lean ground beef
- 1½ cups water, plus 2 tablespoons
- ½ cup sour cream
- 10 tablespoons uncooked brown rice
- 1 large egg yolk
- 3 tablespoons mustard, divided

- Pinch salt
- Pinch freshly ground black pepper
- Olive oil cooking spray

Directions:

1. Warm your oven to 350 F. Spray a 6-cup muffin tin with cooking spray and set aside.
2. Combine the water and brown rice over medium heat in a medium saucepan.
3. Bring to a boil, then reduce the heat, cover, and simmer for 25 to 30 minutes or until the rice is tender. Strain if necessary and set aside to cool within 20 minutes.
4. Meanwhile, combine the ground beef, egg yolk, 1 tablespoon of mustard, salt, and pepper in a medium bowl and mix well.
5. Divide the beef mixture into 5 balls and press into the prepared cups against the

sides and bottom, making a "crust," leaving a space for the filling.

6. Combine the remaining 2 tablespoons of mustard with the sour cream in your small bowl and mix them. Add the sour cream mixture to the rice and mix them.
7. Spoon about ¼ cup of the rice mixture into the center of the beef cups. Put 2 tablespoons of water in the empty muffin cup.
8. Bake the meatloaves for 22 to 27 minutes or until a food thermometer inserted into the center reads 160 F and the juices run clear.
9. Let cool for 5 minutes, unmold and serve.

Nutritional Values: Calories: 344; Total Fat: 14g; Carbohydrates: 19g; Protein: 34g; Fiber: 1g; Phosphorus: 338mg; Potassium: 462mg; Sodium: 210mg; Cholesterol: 147.6mg; Iron 4mg; Vitamin A: 190.8mcg; Vitamin C: 1.5mg

11. Lemon-Butter Tilapia

Preparation Time: 10 minutes

Cooking time: 15 minutes

Servings: 4

Ingredients:

- 8 ounces fresh tilapia
- 3 tablespoons unsalted butter, melted
- 2 tablespoons lemon juice
- 1 teaspoon freshly ground black pepper
- 1 tablespoon garlic powder
- ½ teaspoon red pepper flakes
- ½ teaspoon dried parsley
- 1 lemon, sliced into rounds

Directions:

1. Warm your oven to 400 F. Line a baking sheet using parchment paper.
2. Mix the pepper, butter, garlic powder, red pepper flakes, parsley, and lemon juice in a medium bowl.

3. Place the tilapia on the prepared baking sheet and pour the lemon-butter mixture over the fish to coat. Top with the lemon slices.
4. Bake in the oven within 10 to 12 minutes, until the fish is tender and flaky.

Nutritional Values: Calories: 143; Total Fat: 9.5g; Carbohydrates: 3g; Protein: 12g; Fiber: 0.5g; Phosphorus: 111mg; Potassium: 223mg; Sodium: 33mg; Cholesterol: 59.02mg; Iron 0.9mg; Vitamin A: 100mcg; Vitamin C: 5.4mg

12. Ginger Shrimp with Snow Peas

Preparation Time: 20 minutes

Cooking time: 12 minutes

Servings: 4

Ingredients:

- 1-pound medium shrimp, shelled and deveined

- 2 cups snow peas
- 1½ cups frozen baby peas
- 3 tablespoons water
- 2 tablespoons low-sodium soy sauce
- 2 tablespoons extra-virgin olive oil
- 1 tablespoon minced peeled fresh ginger
- 1/8 teaspoon freshly ground black pepper

Directions:

1. Heat the olive oil in your large skillet over medium heat. Add the ginger and stir-fry for 1 to 2 minutes until the ginger is fragrant.
2. Add the snow peas and stir-fry for 2 to 3 minutes, until they are tender-crisp.
3. Add the baby peas and the water and stir. Cover the skillet and steam for 2 to 3 minutes or until the vegetables are tender.
4. Stir in the shrimp and stir-fry for 3 to 4 minutes, or until the shrimp have curled

and turned pink. Add the soy sauce and pepper; stir and serve.

Nutritional Values: Calories: 237; Total Fat: 7g; Carbohydrates: 12g; Protein: 32g; Fiber: 4g; Phosphorus: 350mg; Potassium: 504mg; Sodium: 469mg; Cholesterol: 59.02mg; Iron 3.6mg; Vitamin A: 256.2mcg; Vitamin C: 21.7mg

13. Red Pepper Pasta

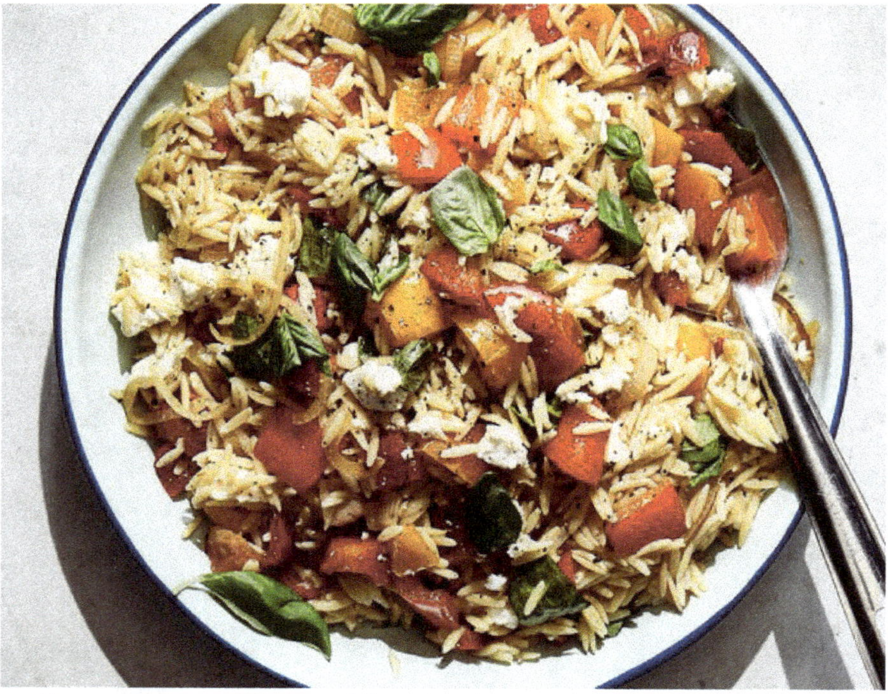

Preparation Time: 10 minutes

Cooking time: 15 minutes

Servings: 4

Ingredients:

- 8 ounces dry orzo pasta
- 2 large red bell peppers, diced
- 2 garlic cloves, minced

- 2 cups Roasted Red Pepper Sauce
- ½ cup halved white button mushrooms
- 4 tablespoons grated Parmesan cheese
- 2 tablespoons olive oil

Directions:

1. Preheat the oven to 42 F. Line a baking sheet with parchment paper.
2. In a medium bowl, combine the bell peppers, mushrooms, olive oil, and garlic and toss together to coat with the olive oil.
3. Transfer the vegetables to the prepared baking sheet and roast in the oven for about 15 minutes or until soft.
4. Cook the pasta as stated in its package directions while the vegetables are roasting.
5. Drain and transfer the pasta to your large bowl. Coat the pasta with the pepper sauce, add the roasted

vegetables, and combine. Top with the Parmesan cheese and serve warm.

Nutritional Values: Calories: 410; Total Fat: Protein: 11g; 13g; Carbohydrates: 61g; Fiber: 6g; Phosphorus: 72mg; Potassium: 445mg; Sodium: 289mg; Cholesterol: 40mg; Iron 2.7mg; Vitamin A: 30mcg; Vitamin C: 5mg

14. Turkey and Corn Chowder

Preparation Time: 20 minutes

Cooking time: 35 minutes

Servings: 6

Ingredients:

- 2 cups shredded cooked turkey or chicken
- 2 russet potatoes, peeled and chopped
- 1 onion, chopped
- 4 cups water
- 1½ cups frozen yellow corn
- 1 cup heavy cream

- 2 tablespoons extra-virgin olive oil
- 1/8 teaspoon salt
- 1/8 teaspoon freshly ground black pepper

Directions:

1. Place the potatoes in your large saucepan, cover with water, and bring to a boil on high heat. Boil for 10 minutes, then drain the potatoes and discard the water.
2. In your large saucepan, heat the olive oil over medium heat. Add the onion and cook for 3 to 4 minutes, stirring until tender.
3. Add the water, corn, potatoes, salt, and pepper and bring to a simmer.
4. Adjust the heat to low and simmer within 20 to 25 minutes or until the potatoes are tender. Remove half the vegetables from the soup and puree. Return to the soup.

5. Add the turkey and cream to the soup. Heat over medium heat until steaming; do not boil. Serve.

Nutritional Values: Calories: 307; Total Fat: 20g; Carbohydrates: 16g; Protein: 17g; Fiber: 2g; Phosphorus: 181mg; Potassium: 407mg; Sodium: 110mg; Cholesterol: 31mg; Iron 3.5mg; Vitamin A: 186mcg; Vitamin C: 27.2mg

15. Spinach Alfredo Lasagna Rolls

Preparation Time: 25 minutes

Cooking time: 50 minutes

Servings: 4

Ingredients:

- 4 whole-grain lasagna noodles
- 2 cups frozen whole-leaf spinach, thawed (measure while frozen)
- 1 large onion, chopped

- 1 (8-oz) package cream cheese, warm, divided
- 1/3 cup shredded Parmesan cheese
- 2 tablespoons extra-virgin olive oil

Directions:

1. Let your large pot filled with water comes to a boil over high heat, and add the lasagna noodles.
2. Simmer for 8 to 9 minutes or until the pasta is almost al dente but still has a thin white line in the center. Drain, reserving ¼ cup of the pasta water, and set aside.
3. Meanwhile, in your saucepan, heat the olive oil over medium heat. Add the onions and cook for 6 to 8 minutes, stirring, until the onions are tender and starting to turn brown.
4. While the onions are cooking, drain the spinach and put the leaves into paper

towels. Squeeze well to remove most of the water from the spinach.

5. Add the spinach to the onions, stir, and turn off the heat. Add 6 ounces of cream cheese to the vegetables and stir until combined. Set aside.
6. Combine the remaining 2 ounces of cream cheese in a small saucepan with the reserved pasta water. Heat over low heat, often stirring with a wire whisk, until smooth.
7. In a 9-inch baking dish, place 2 tablespoons of the cream cheese sauce.
8. On a work surface, place the lasagna noodles. Divide the spinach mixture among them and roll them up.
9. Place the rolls, seam-side down, on the sauce in the casserole. Top with the remaining sauce.
10. Sprinkle the lasagna rolls with the Parmesan cheese. Bake within 25 to 35

minutes, until the lasagna is bubbling and the top starts to brown.

Nutritional Values: Calories: 388; Total Fat: 24g; Carbohydrates: 34g; Protein: 13g; Fiber: 9g; Phosphorus: 119mg; Potassium: 378mg; Sodium: 411mg; Cholesterol: 159.5mg; Iron 2.8mg; Vitamin A: 943mcg; Vitamin C: 9.2mg

16. Crustless Cabbage Quiche

Preparation Time: 10 minutes

Cooking time: 40 minutes

Servings: 6

Ingredients:

- 3 large eggs, beaten
- 3 large egg whites, beaten
- 3 cups coleslaw blend with carrots
- 1 cup grated Swiss cheese
- ½ cup half-and-half
- 2 tablespoons extra-virgin olive oil
- 1 teaspoon dried dill weed

- 1/8 teaspoon salt
- 1/8 teaspoon freshly ground black pepper
- Olive oil cooking spray

Directions:

1. Warm your oven to 350 F. Spray a 9-inch pie plate with cooking spray and set aside.
2. In a large skillet, heat the olive oil over medium heat. Add the coleslaw mix and cook for 4 to 6 minutes, stirring, until the cabbage is tender.
3. Transfer the vegetables from the pan to a medium bowl to cool.
4. Meanwhile, mix the eggs and egg whites, half-and-half, dill, salt, and pepper in your separate medium bowl and beat to combine.
5. Stir the cabbage mixture into the egg mixture and pour it into the prepared pie plate. Sprinkle with the cheese.

6. Bake within 30 to 35 minutes, or until the mixture is puffed, set, and light golden brown. Let stand within 5 minutes, then slice to serve.

Nutritional Values: Calories: 203; Total Fat: 16g; Carbohydrates: 5g; Protein: 11g; Fiber: 1g; Phosphorus: 169mg; Potassium: 155mg; Sodium: 321mg; Cholesterol: 225mg; Iron 4mg; Vitamin A: 433.8mcg; Vitamin C: 46mg

17. White Bean Veggie Burgers

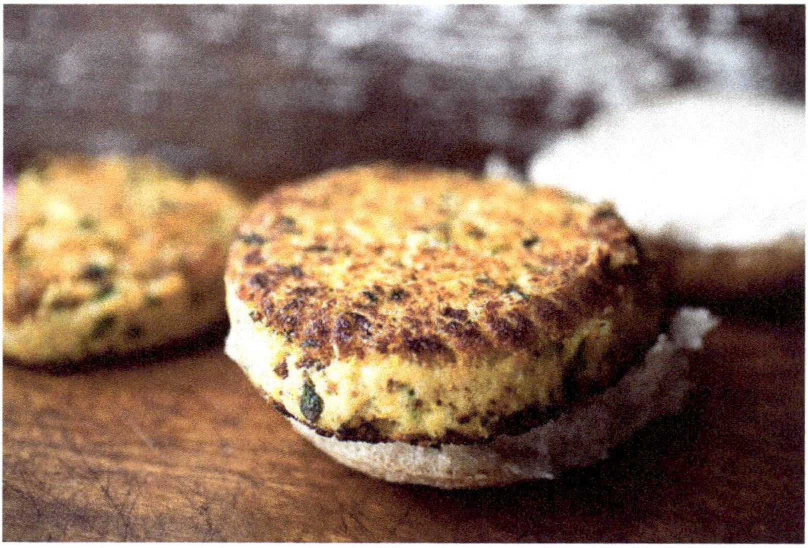

Preparation Time: 10 minutes

Cooking time: 15 minutes

Servings: 4

Ingredients:

- 1 cup canned white beans, drained & rinsed
- 1 cup cooked white rice
- 1 large egg
- ½ cup fresh or frozen corn
- 1 teaspoon garlic powder

- ½ sweet onion, finely chopped
- ½ cup red bell pepper, finely chopped
- 1/3 cup all-purpose flour
- 2 teaspoons extra-virgin olive oil
- 2 teaspoons dried thyme
- ½ teaspoon ground chipotle pepper
- Juice of 1 lemon
- Freshly ground black pepper, as needed

Directions:

1. In your large bowl, mash the beans with a potato masher, leaving a few whole beans as desired.
2. Add the rice, garlic powder, thyme, chipotle pepper, onion, corn, bell pepper, lemon, flour, and egg, and mix well to blend—season with pepper.
3. Using your hands, form the mixture into four patties.
4. In your large skillet over medium heat, heat the olive oil. Cook the burgers for 5 minutes until browned on one side, flip,

and cook the other side for an additional 5 minutes. Serve and enjoy!

Nutritional Values: Calories: 305; Total Fat: 4g; Carbohydrates: 57g; Protein: 11g; Fiber: 6g; Phosphorus: 181mg; Potassium: 515mg; Sodium: 281mg; Cholesterol: 0mg; Iron 3mg; Vitamin A: 74.4mcg; Vitamin C: 1mg

18. Baked Herbed Chicken

Preparation Time: 10 minutes

Cooking time: 40 minutes

Servings: 6

Ingredients:

- 6 bone-in chicken thighs
- 4 tablespoons butter, at room temperature
- 4 garlic cloves, minced
- 1 tablespoon chopped fresh oregano
- 1 tablespoon chopped fresh parsley
- 1 teaspoon lemon zest

- ¼ teaspoon freshly ground black pepper

Directions:

1. Preheat the oven to 425 F.
2. Add the butter, garlic, oregano, parsley, and lemon zest in your small bowl. Mix well. Keep aside.
3. Arrange the thighs on a baking tray and gently peel back the skin, leaving it attached.
4. Brush the thigh meat with a couple of teaspoons of the butter mixture, and replace the skin to cover the meat. Season with pepper.
5. Bake within 40 minutes until the skin is crisp and the juices run clear. Let it rest within 5 minutes before serving.

Nutritional Values: Calories: 226; Total Fat: 17g; Carbohydrates: 1g; Protein: 16g; Fiber: 0g; Phosphorus: 114mg; Potassium: 158mg;

Sodium: 120mg; Cholesterol: 78mg; Iron 0.8mg; Vitamin A: 40.5mcg; Vitamin C: 2.6mg

19. White Fish and Broccoli Curry

Preparation Time: 10 minutes

Cooking time: 10 minutes

Servings: 6

Ingredients:

For the curry paste:

- ½ sweet onion, chopped
- 1 medium red chile, chopped
- 1 lemongrass stalk, outer leaves removed, tender bottom portion chopped
- 1-inch piece ginger, peeled and chopped
- ¼ cup roughly chopped fresh cilantro stems
- 2 tablespoons extra-virgin olive oil
- 1 teaspoon turmeric powder
- ½ teaspoon cumin seeds

For the curry:

- 1 pound tilapia fillets
- 3 cups broccoli florets
- ¾ cup unsweetened store-bought rice milk or almond milk
- ½ cup cream cheese
- Juice of 1 lime
- 1 teaspoon sugar

Directions:

1. Using a mortar, pestle, or blender, combine the onion, chile, ginger, lemongrass, cilantro, turmeric, cumin seeds, and olive oil, and blend until smooth.
2. In your large skillet over medium-high heat, heat the curry paste, and cook, occasionally stirring, until fragrant for 2 to 3 minutes. Add the rice milk and stir until incorporated. Bring to a light simmer.
3. Meanwhile, in a small bowl, add the cream cheese. Add a few tablespoons of

the hot rice-milk mixture and stir until blended.

4. Add the tilapia and broccoli to the skillet, then add the cream cheese mixture, gently stirring to blend.
5. Cook for 3 to 5 minutes, until the fish is cooked through, the broccoli is fork-tender, and the curry is bubbly.
6. Stir in the lime juice and sugar. Remove from the heat, and serve over white rice.

Nutritional Values: Calories: 223; Total Fat: 13g; Carbohydrates: 10g; Protein: 18g; Fiber: 2g; Phosphorus: 194mg; Potassium: 490mg; Sodium: 134mg; Cholesterol: 56mg; Iron 1mg; Vitamin A: 531.3mcg; Vitamin C: 2mg

20. Pepper Jack and Rice Stuffed Peppers

Preparation Time: 20 minutes

Cooking time: 1 hour & 5 minutes

Servings: 4

Ingredients:

- 6 red bell peppers, divided (4 top cut off & seed removed & 2 seeded & chopped)
- 1 onion, chopped
- 2 cups cooked brown rice
- 2/3 cup shredded pepper jack cheese
- 2 tablespoons extra-virgin olive oil
- ½ teaspoon Italian seasoning
- 1/8 teaspoon salt
- 1/8 teaspoon freshly ground black pepper

Directions:

1. Warm your oven to 375 F.
2. In your large saucepan, heat the olive oil over medium heat. Add the onion and cook within 3 minutes, stirring, until crisp-tender.
3. Add the chopped bell peppers. Sprinkle with Italian seasoning, salt, and pepper—Cook and stir for 3 to 5 minutes or until

crisp-tender. Stir in the brown rice and remove from the heat.

4. Stir the cheese into the vegetable mixture. Place the bell peppers into a casserole dish, so they fit snugly. Fill each pepper with the vegetable mixture.
5. Pour ½ cup of water into the casserole dish, around the bell peppers. Cover the dish with aluminum foil.
6. Bake for 35 minutes, then remove the foil. Bake for another 20 to 25 minutes or until the peppers are tender and the filling is brown on top.

Nutritional Values: Calories: 316; Total Fat: 14g; Carbohydrates: 40g; Protein: 9g; Fiber: 6g; Phosphorus: 249mg; Potassium: 580mg; Sodium: 202mg; Cholesterol: 64mg; Iron 1.76mg; Vitamin A: 25mcg; Vitamin C: 40.8mg

21. Meatloaf with Mushroom Gravy

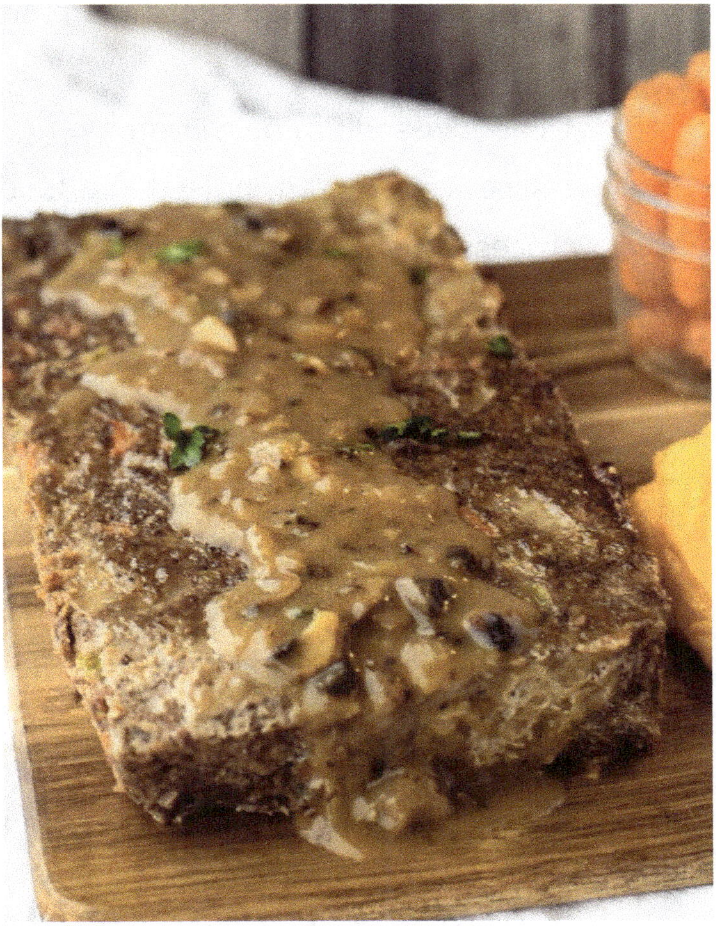

Preparation Time: 10 minutes

Cooking time: 50 minutes

Servings: 8

Ingredients:

- 1½ pounds lean ground beef
- 1 (8-ounce) package sliced cremini mushrooms
- 1 cup low-sodium beef broth
- 1 slice white bread, pulsed in a food processor into coarse bread crumbs
- 1 sweet onion, finely chopped
- 1 large egg
- 3 garlic cloves, minced
- 1 tbsp +1 tsp olive oil, divided
- 1 teaspoon dried oregano
- 1 tablespoon all-purpose flour
- ¼ teaspoon freshly ground black pepper
- Nonstick cooking spray

Directions:

1. Warm your oven to 350 F. Coat a loaf pan with nonstick cooking spray.
2. In your large skillet over medium-high heat, heat 1 tablespoon of olive oil. Add the mushrooms and oregano. Cook for 5 minutes, stirring occasionally.

3. Add the onion and garlic, and continue to cook for 5 minutes, until the mushrooms and onion are soft. Remove from the heat.
4. Divide the mushroom mixture into two equal parts and finely chop one part. Set the other part aside.
5. Add the chopped mushroom mixture, beef, egg, bread crumbs, and pepper in a medium bowl. Mix well.
6. Form the beef mixture into a loaf and transfer it into the loaf pan. Bake for 45 minutes until cooked through.
7. Heat the rest of the 1 tsp of olive oil in your saucepan over medium-high heat, and add the remaining mushroom mixture.
8. Stir in the flour and mix until coated. Slowly add the broth, constantly stirring to break up any clumps. Bring to a boil, reduce the heat, and simmer for 5 minutes until thickened.

9. Spoon the gravy over slices of meatloaf, and serve.

Nutritional Values: Calories: 280; Total Fat: 20g; Carbohydrates: 7g; Protein: 17g; Fiber: 1g; Phosphorus: 192mg; Potassium: 394mg; Sodium: 146mg; Cholesterol: 100mg; Iron 2.7mg; Vitamin A: 90mcg; Vitamin C: 30mg

22. Chicken, Pasta, and Broccoli Bake

Preparation Time: 10 minutes

Cooking time: 30 minutes

Servings: 6

Ingredients:

- 8 ounces egg noodles
- 3 cups shredded cooked chicken breast
- 1 (10-ounce) package broccoli florets
- ½ sweet onion, chopped
- 1½ cups low-sodium chicken stock

- ¾ cup unsweetened store-bought rice milk or almond milk
- ¼ cup shredded Cheddar cheese
- ¼ cup all-purpose flour
- 2 tablespoons butter
- Freshly ground black pepper, as needed

Directions:

1. Warm your oven to 350 F. Grease a 2-quart baking dish.
2. Fill a large pot with water and bring to a boil. Add the egg noodles and cook for 5 minutes.
3. Add the broccoli, then continue to cook within 3 to 5 more minutes, until the noodles are tender and the broccoli is just fork-tender. Drain and set aside.
4. In your medium saucepan over medium-high heat, heat the butter. Add the onion and cook for 3 to 5 minutes until it softens.

5. Add the flour, then stir until evenly mixed. Add the broth and season with pepper. Simmer for 5 minutes until it begins to thicken. Add the rice milk and cook until heated through.
6. Toss the sauce with the broccoli, noodles, and cooked chicken, and transfer to the prepared baking dish. Top with the Cheddar cheese.
7. Bake for 20 minutes, uncovered until browned and bubbly. Serve and enjoy!

Nutritional Values: Calories: 351; Total Fat: 11g; Carbohydrates: 38g; Protein: 24g; Fiber: 3g; Phosphorus: 271mg; Potassium: 402mg; Sodium: 152mg; Cholesterol: 42mg; Iron 3mg; Vitamin A: 249.3mcg; Vitamin C: 92mg

23. Pineapple-Soy Salmon Stir-Fry

Preparation Time: 15 minutes

Cooking time: 15 minutes

Servings: 4

Ingredients:

- 1 (8-ounce) can crushed pineapple, strained, reserving juice
- 2 tablespoons low-sodium soy sauce
- 1 tablespoon cornstarch
- 1/8 teaspoon freshly ground black pepper
- 2 tablespoons extra-virgin olive oil
- 2 (6-ounce) salmon fillets without skin, cubed
- 1 (16-ounce) bag frozen stir-fry vegetables

Directions:

1. Whisk the reserved pineapple juice, soy sauce, cornstarch, and pepper in a small bowl and set aside.
2. In your large skillet, heat the olive oil. Add the salmon cubes and stir-fry for 3 to 4 minutes, or until the salmon flakes with a fork.

3. Transfer the salmon to a plate and set aside using a slotted spoon.
4. Add the frozen vegetables to the skillet. Stir-fry for another 3 to 4 minutes, or until the vegetables are hot and tender. Return the salmon to the skillet and add the pineapple.
5. Whisk the sauce again and add to the skillet; stir-fry for 3 to 4 minutes or until the sauce bubbles and has thickened. Serve.

Nutritional Values: Calories: 280; Total Fat: 13g; Carbohydrates: 21g; Protein: 22g; Fiber: 3g; Phosphorus: 271mg; Potassium: 599mg; Sodium: 361mg; Cholesterol: 78mg; Iron 1.6mg; Vitamin A: 29.1mcg; Vitamin C: 14.8mg

24. Mediterranean Eggplant Casserole

Preparation Time: 10 minutes

Cooking time: 50 minutes

Servings: 4

Ingredients:

- 2 large eggplants, sliced into ½-inch pieces (8 cups)
- 2 garlic cloves, minced
- 1 medium green bell pepper, diced
- 1 large white onion, diced
- 1 cup canned tomatoes, diced, no added salt
- ¼ cup shredded part-skim mozzarella cheese
- 3 tablespoons olive oil, divided
- 3 tablespoons dried parsley
- 1 tablespoon dried thyme
- 1 tablespoon all-purpose flour

Directions:

1. Warm your oven to 375 F. Coat a casserole dish with 1½ tablespoons of olive oil.

2. Heat the remaining 1½ tablespoons of olive oil in a large skillet and sauté the onion until tender, about 10 minutes. Add the garlic and bell pepper and cook for about 3 minutes.
3. Add the tomatoes, parsley, and thyme and simmer for a few minutes. Transfer the mixture to a bowl and set aside.
4. In the same skillet, add the eggplant, frequently stirring until browned, about 5 minutes. Add the flour and stir. Add the tomato mixture and bring to a simmer.
5. Spoon half of the vegetable mixture into your prepared casserole dish. Top with 1/8 cup of mozzarella cheese.
6. Add the remaining vegetables and top with the remaining 1/8 cup of mozzarella cheese—Bake for about 30 minutes, or until the cheese is bubbly.

Nutritional Values: Calories: 202; Protein: 5g; Total Fat: 12g; Carbohydrates: 20g; Fiber:

6.5g; Phosphorus: 106mg; Potassium: 680mg; Sodium: 71mg; Cholesterol: 137.5mg; Iron 7.6mg; Vitamin A: 29.2mcg; Vitamin C: 17.9mg

25. Mediterranean Cod

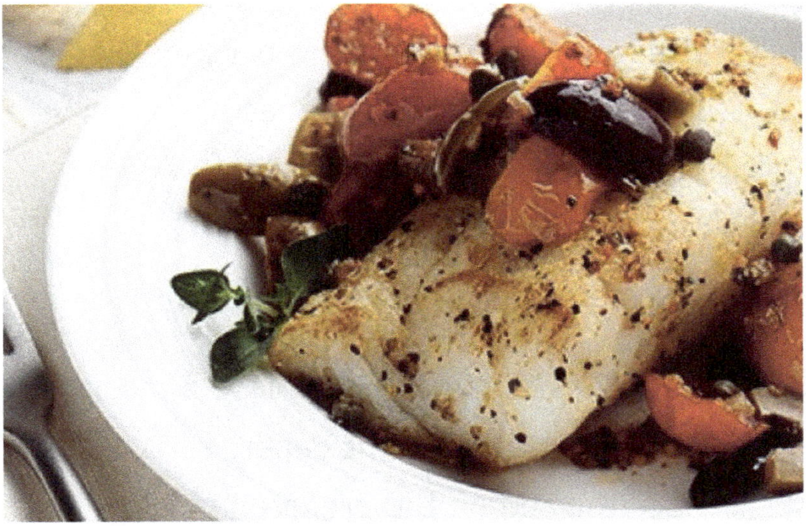

Preparation Time: 10 minutes

Cooking time: 20 minutes

Servings: 4

Ingredients:

- 8 ounces skinless fresh cod

- 4 leeks, chopped white & light green parts
- 2 Roma tomatoes, quartered
- 1 medium green bell pepper, quartered
- 1 medium white onion, quartered
- 2 tablespoons olive oil
- 1 teaspoon freshly ground black pepper
- 1 teaspoon red pepper flakes
- 1 teaspoon dried parsley
- 1 teaspoon garlic powder

Directions:

1. Warm your oven to 425 F. Line a baking sheet using parchment paper.
2. Place the cod on the prepared baking sheet and arrange the bell pepper, tomatoes, onion, and leeks around it.
3. Combine the olive oil, pepper, red pepper flakes, parsley, and garlic powder in a small bowl. Drizzle over the fish and vegetables on the baking sheet.

4. Bake in the oven for about 20 minutes, or until the fish is flaky, tender, and no longer translucent.

Nutritional Values: Calories: 183; Protein: 11g; Total Fat: 7.5g; Carbohydrates: 19g; Fiber: 3.5g; Phosphorus: 112mg; Potassium: 451mg; Sodium: 53mg; Cholesterol: 48.8mg; Iron 1mg; Vitamin A: 380.1mcg; Vitamin C: 21.1mg

SNACKS

26. Cinnamon Apple Chips

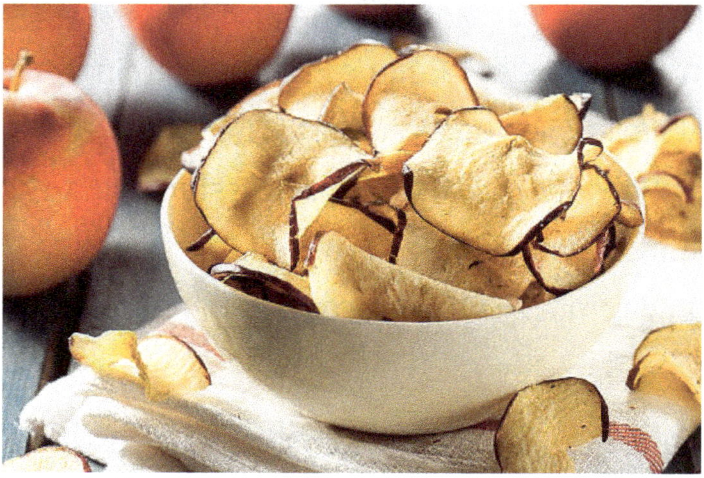

Preparation Time: 10 minutes

Cooking time: 2-3 hours

Servings: 4

Ingredients:

- 4 apples
- 1 teaspoon ground cinnamon

Directions:

1. Warm your oven to 200 F. Line a baking sheet using parchment paper. Core the apples and cut them into 1/8-inch slices.
2. In a medium bowl, toss the apple slices with the cinnamon. Spread the apples in a single layer on the prepared baking sheet.
3. Cook for 2 to 3 hours until the apples are dry. They will still be soft while hot but will crisp once completely cooled. Store in an airtight container for up to four days.

Nutritional Values: Calories: 96; Total Fat: 0g; Carbohydrates: 26g; Protein: 1g; Fiber: 5g; Phosphorus: 0mg; Potassium: 198mg; Sodium: 2mg; Cholesterol: 0mg; Iron 0mg; Vitamin A: 0mcg; Vitamin C: 18mg

27. Parmesan Roasted Cauliflower

Preparation Time: 15 minutes

Cooking time: 25 minutes

Servings: 4

Ingredients:

- 4 cups cauliflower florets
- ½ cup grated Parmesan cheese
- 2 tablespoons extra-virgin olive oil
- 4 garlic cloves, minced
- ½ teaspoon dried thyme leaves
- ¼ teaspoon freshly ground black pepper
- 1/8 teaspoon salt

Directions:

1. Preheat the oven to 400 F.
2. On a baking sheet, combine the cauliflower, Parmesan cheese, olive oil, garlic, thyme, pepper, and salt and toss to coat.
3. Roast within 25 to 30 minutes, stirring once during cooking time, until the cauliflower has light golden-brown edges and is tender. Serve.

Nutritional Values: Calories: 144; Total Fat: 11g; Carbohydrates: 4g; Protein: 6g; Fiber: 1g; Phosphorus: 130mg; Potassium: 359mg; Sodium: 332mg; Cholesterol: 2mg; Iron 0.73mg; Vitamin A: 4mcg; Vitamin C: 72.6mg

28. Baba Ghanoush Dip

Preparation Time: 10 minutes

Cooking time: 30 minutes

Servings: 8

Ingredients:

- 2 medium eggplants, halved
- 2 garlic cloves
- ¼ teaspoon ground cumin
- ¼ teaspoon paprika
- 1 tablespoon lemon juice

Directions:

1. Warm your oven to 400 F. Roast the eggplants for about 30 minutes, or until

the interior is very tender and the skin is collapsing and a deep dark purple.
2. Scoop out the flesh of the eggplants with a large spoon, leaving the skin behind.
3. In a high-speed blender or food processor, combine the eggplant flesh, garlic, cumin, paprika, and lemon juice and mix until smooth. Serve immediately.

Nutritional Values: Calories: 36; Total Fat: 0g; Carbohydrates: 8g; Protein: 1g; Fiber: 4g; Phosphorus: 34mg; Potassium: 320mg; Sodium: 3mg; Cholesterol: 0mg; Iron 0.4mg; Vitamin A: 0mcg; Vitamin C: 48mg

29. Fruit Dip

Preparation Time: 10 minutes

Cooking time: 0 minutes

Servings: 2 cups

Ingredients:

- 1 cup plain cream cheese, softened
- 1 cup plain low-fat probiotic yogurt
- 1 teaspoon vanilla extract
- 1 tablespoon lemon juice
- 1 tablespoon ground cinnamon
- Cut fruit of your choice for serving

Directions:

1. In your blender or food processor, mix the cream cheese, yogurt, vanilla, lemon juice, and cinnamon until well combined.
2. Place the cream cheese mixture in a small bowl and chill, covered, in the refrigerator for 45 minutes. Remove and serve with the fruit of your choice.

Nutritional Values: Calories: 97; Total Fat: 7g; Carbohydrates: 7g; Protein: 2g; Fiber: 1g; Phosphorus: 54mg; Potassium: 97mg; Sodium: 75mg; Cholesterol: 9.2mg; Iron 0mg; Vitamin A: 28.1mcg; Vitamin C: 0.3mg

30. Baked Jicama Fries

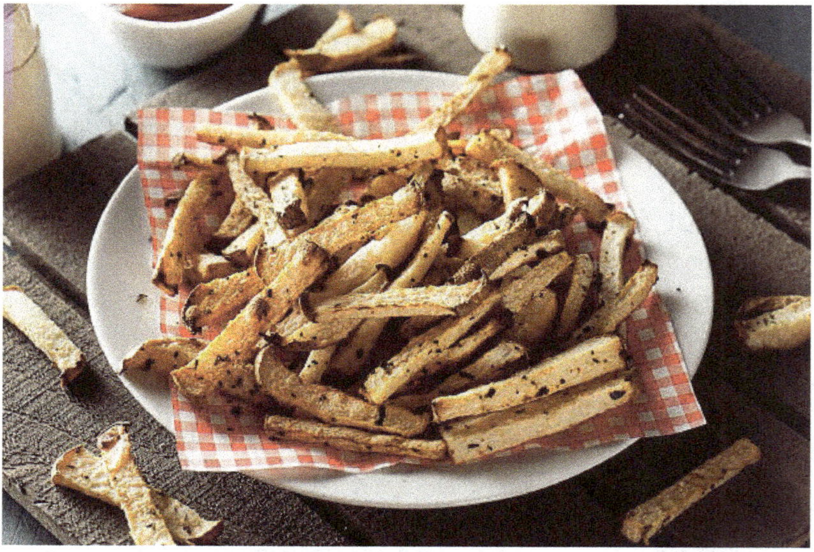

Preparation Time: 20 minutes

Cooking time: 50 minutes

Servings: 4

Ingredients:

- 1 pound jicama root
- 2 tablespoons butter
- 2 tablespoons grated Parmesan cheese
- 1 tablespoon extra-virgin olive oil
- 1 teaspoon chili powder

- 1 teaspoon paprika
- ¼ teaspoon salt
- 1/8 teaspoon freshly ground black pepper

Directions:

1. Peel the jicama and cut it into ½-inch slices. Cut the slices into strips, each about 4 inches long.
2. In a large saucepan, place the jicama strips and cover them with water. Bring to a boil, then boil for 9 minutes.
3. Drain the jicama well and transfer to a rimmed baking sheet. Pat the strips using a paper towel until they are dry to a crisp in the oven. Preheat the oven to 400 F.
4. In your small saucepan, melt the butter with olive oil. Drizzle over the jicama on the baking sheet.

5. Sprinkle with the chili powder, paprika, salt, and pepper and toss to coat. Spread the strips into a single layer.
6. Bake the jicama fries for 40 to 45 minutes or until they are browned and crisp, turning once with a spatula halfway through the cooking time. Sprinkle with the Parmesan cheese and serve.

Nutritional Values: Calories: 140; Total Fat: 10g; Carbohydrates: 11g; Protein: 2g; Fiber: 6g; Phosphorus: 45mg; Potassium: 204mg; Sodium: 273mg; Cholesterol: 0mg; Iron 0.6mg; Vitamin A: 60mcg; Vitamin C: 16.2mg

31. Savory Collard Chips

Preparation Time: 5 minutes

Cooking time: 20 minutes

Servings: 4

Ingredients:

- 1 bunch collard greens
- 1 teaspoon extra-virgin olive oil
- Juice of ½ lemon
- ½ teaspoon garlic powder
- ¼ teaspoon freshly ground black pepper

Directions:

1. Warm your oven to 350 F. Line a baking sheet using parchment paper.
2. Cut the collards into 2-by-2-inch squares and pat dry with paper towels.
3. Toss the greens with olive oil, lemon juice, garlic powder, and pepper in a large bowl. Use your hands to mix well, massaging the dressing into the greens until evenly coated.
4. Arrange the collards in a single layer on the baking sheet, and cook for 8 minutes. Flip the pieces and cook for an additional 8 minutes, until crisp.

5. Remove from the oven, let cool, and store in an airtight container in a cool location for up to three days.

Nutritional Values: Calories: 24; Total Fat: 1g; Carbohydrates: 3g; Protein: 1g; Fiber: 1g; Phosphorus: 6mg; Potassium: 72mg; Sodium: 8mg; Cholesterol: 3mg; Iron 0.65mg; Vitamin A: 83.2mcg; Vitamin C: 8.5mg

32. Roasted Red Pepper Hummus

Preparation Time: 10 minutes

Cooking time: 10 minutes

Servings: 8

Ingredients:

- 1 red bell pepper
- 1 (15-ounce) can chickpeas, drained and rinsed
- Juice of 1 lemon
- 2 tablespoons tahini
- 2 garlic cloves

- 2 tablespoons extra-virgin olive oil

Directions:

1. Set an oven rack to the highest part. Heat the broiler to high.
2. Core the pepper and cut it into three or four large pieces. Arrange them on a baking sheet, skin-side up.
3. Broil the peppers for 5 to 10 minutes until the skins are charred. Remove from the oven and transfer the peppers to a small bowl.
4. Cover using plastic wrap and let them steam for 10 to 15 minutes, until cool enough to handle.
5. Peel the charred skin off the peppers, and place the peppers in a blender.
6. Add the chickpeas, lemon juice, tahini, garlic, and olive oil. Process until smooth, adding up to 1 tablespoon of water to adjust consistency as desired.

Nutritional Values: Calories: 103; Total Fat: 6g; Carbohydrates: 10g; Protein: 3g; Fiber: 3g; Phosphorus: 58mg; Potassium: 91mg; Sodium: 72mg; Cholesterol: 0mg; Iron 0.7mg; Vitamin A: 5mcg; Vitamin C: 0mg

33. Roasted Onion Dip

Preparation Time: 15 minutes

Cooking time: 35 minutes

Servings: 1 ½ cup

Ingredients:

- 1 red onion, chopped
- 2 tablespoons extra-virgin olive oil
- 1 (8-ounce) package cream cheese, at room temperature
- 2 tablespoons mayonnaise (made with avocado oil or olive oil)
- 1 tablespoon freshly squeezed lemon juice
- ½ teaspoon dried thyme leaves

Directions:

1. Preheat the oven to 400 F. Combine the onion and olive oil on a rimmed baking sheet and toss to coat.
2. Roast for 30 to 35 minutes, occasionally stirring, until the onions are soft and golden brown. Don't let them burn. Transfer to a plate and set aside.
3. Beat the cream cheese, mayonnaise, lemon juice, and thyme leaves in your medium bowl. Stir in the onions.
4. Cover and refrigerate it for up to 8 hours before serving.

Nutritional Values: Calories: 212; Total Fat: 21g; Carbohydrates: 4g; Protein: 3g; Fiber: 0g; Phosphorus: 47mg; Potassium: 82mg; Sodium: 149mg; Cholesterol: 15mg; Iron 0mg; Vitamin A: 18mcg; Vitamin C: 0mg

34. Honey-Vanilla Energy Balls

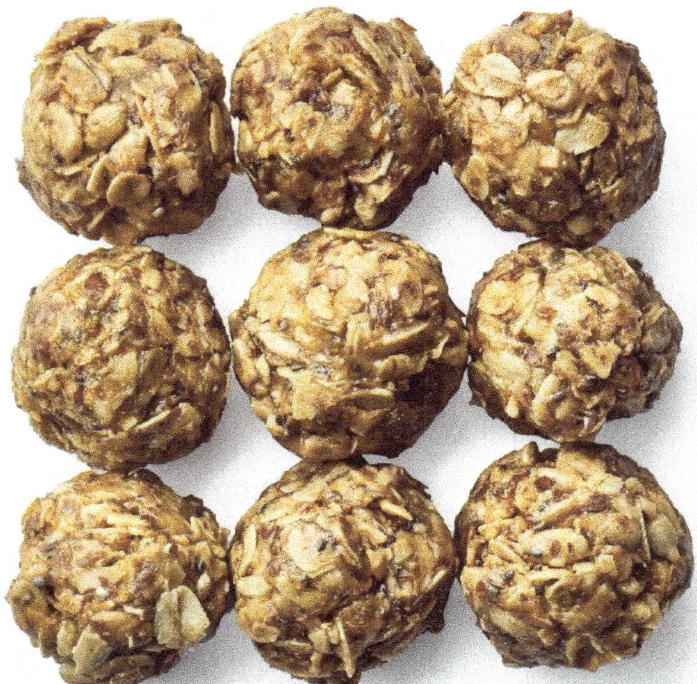

Preparation Time: 10 minutes + chilling time

Cooking time: 0 minutes

Servings: 20 balls

Ingredients:

- 1½ cups old-fashioned rolled oats
- ½ cup unsalted peanut butter
- ¼ cup honey
- 1½ teaspoons vanilla extract
- 2 tablespoons chia seeds

Directions:

1. Line a pan or baking sheet, using parchment paper.
2. Combine the oats, peanut butter, honey, vanilla, and chia seeds in a large bowl.
3. Roll into 20 balls approximately 1 inch in diameter each, and place on the prepared baking sheet. Chill for 1 hour in the refrigerator.

Nutritional Values: Calories: 318; Total Fat: 16g; carbohydrates: 37g; Protein: 9g; Fiber: 5g; Phosphorus: 213mg; Potassium: 260mg; Sodium: 6mgg; Cholesterol: 1mg; Iron 1mg; Vitamin A: 21.3mcg; Vitamin C: 0mg

35. Spicy Buffalo Cauliflower Bites

Preparation Time: 10 minutes

Cooking time: 40 minutes

Servings: 12 cauli bites

Ingredients:

- ½ cup water
- ½ cup all-purpose flour
- 2 tablespoons garlic powder
- 1 teaspoon freshly ground black pepper
- 1 small cauliflower head, cut into bite-size pieces
- ¼ cup buffalo hot sauce
- ¾ cup your favorite dipping sauce

Directions:

1. Warm your oven to 450 F. Line a baking sheet using parchment paper.
2. Combine the water, flour, garlic powder, and pepper in a medium bowl and stir well until combined.

3. Coat the cauliflower pieces in the flour mixture. Place on the prepared baking sheet and roast in the oven, tossing halfway through the cooking, for about 20 minutes, or until the bites are golden brown and crunchy.
4. Remove the cauliflower from your oven, place it in a large bowl, and toss to coat with the hot sauce.
5. Place the cauliflower back on your baking sheet and continue baking for 15 to 20 minutes, until crispy.
6. Remove the cauliflower from the oven and sit for 10 minutes before serving. Serve warm with your favorite dipping sauce.

Nutritional Values: Calories: 34; Total Fat: 0.5g; Carbohydrates: 7g; Protein: 1g; Fiber: 1g; Phosphorus: 24mg; Potassium: 102mg; Sodium: 20mg; Cholesterol: 15mg; Iron

0.8mg; Vitamin A: 52.5mcg; Vitamin C: 12.9mg

36. Roasted Garlic White Bean Dip

Preparation Time: 20 minutes

Cooking time: 60 minutes

Servings: 2 cups

Ingredients:

- 1 (15-ounce) can no-salt-added cannellini beans, drained and rinsed
- 2 onions, cut into 8 wedges each
- 2 garlic heads, whole
- ¼ cup extra-virgin olive oil, divided
- 2 tablespoons freshly squeezed lemon juice
- 1 teaspoon dried marjoram leaves
- 1/8 teaspoon salt
- 1/8 teaspoon freshly ground black pepper

Directions:

1. Preheat the oven to 375 F. On a rimmed baking sheet, place the onions.
2. Cut the top inch off each garlic head, just enough to expose the cloves, and discard the top. Place the garlic on the baking sheet with the exposed cloves facing up.
3. Drizzle 1 tablespoon of olive oil directly into the garlic heads, wrap each head in aluminum foil and place back on the baking sheet. Drizzle the onions with another 1 tablespoon of olive oil.
4. Roast the vegetables for 45 to 55 minutes, stirring the onions once during cooking, until the onions are golden brown and the garlic is brown and soft.
5. Remove the foil from the garlic and let the garlic and onions cool for 30 minutes.
6. Combine the cannellini beans, lemon juice, marjoram, salt, and pepper in your blender. Add the onions. Add the garlic cloves to the blender.

7. Blend or process the mixture, drizzling in the remaining 2 tablespoons of olive oil until it is mostly smooth, with some texture. Cover and chill for a few hours before serving.

Nutritional Values: Calories: 166; Total Fat: 10g; Carbohydrates: 17g; Protein: 4g; Fiber: 4g; Phosphorus: 81mg; Potassium: 241mg; Sodium: 74mg; Cholesterol: 0mg; Iron 2mg; Vitamin A: 31.2mcg; Vitamin C: 5mg

37. Cucumbers with Sour Cream

Preparation time: 10 minutes

Cooking time: 0 minutes

Servings: 4

Ingredients:

- 2 medium cucumbers, peeled and sliced thinly
- ½ medium sweet onion, sliced
- ¼ cup white wine vinegar

- 1 tbsp canola oil
- 1/8 tsp black pepper
- ½ cup reduced-fat sour cream

Directions:

1. Toss in cucumber, onion, and other ingredients in a medium-sized bowl.
2. Mix well and refrigerate for 2 hours. Toss again and serve to enjoy.

Nutritional Values: Calories: 64; Total Fat: 5 g; Carbohydrates: 4 g; Protein: 1 g; Fiber: 0.8 g; Potassium: 113 mg; Phosphorus: 24 mg; Sodium: 72 mg; Cholesterol: 3mg; Iron 0.26mg; Vitamin A: 14mcg; Vitamin C: 4.7mg

38. Sweet Savory Meatballs

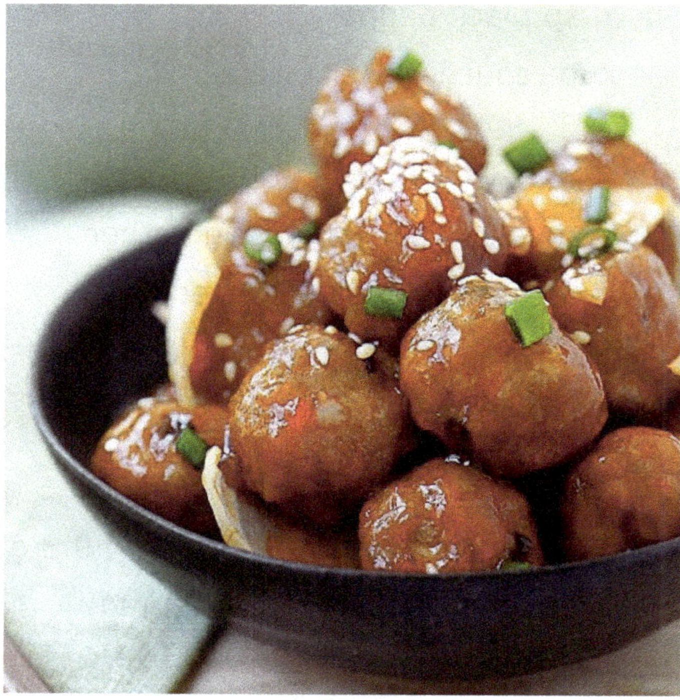

Preparation time: 10 minutes

Cooking time: 20 minutes

Servings: 12

Ingredients:

- 1 lb. ground turkey
- 1 large egg
- ¼ cup breadcrumbs

- 2 tbsp onion, finely chopped
- 1 tsp garlic powder
- ½ tsp black pepper
- ¼ cup canola oil
- 6 oz. grape jelly
- ¼ cup chili sauce

Directions:

1. Place all ingredients except chili sauce and jelly in a large mixing bowl. Mix well until evenly mixed, then make small balls out of this mixture.
2. Spread them out on a greased pan on a stovetop. Cook them over medium heat until brown on all the sides.
3. Mix chili sauce with jelly in a microwave-safe bowl and heat it for 2 minutes in the microwave. Pour this chili sauce mixture onto the meatballs in the pan.
4. Transfer the meatballs in the pan to the preheated oven. Bake the meatballs for

20 minutes in an oven at 375 F. Serve fresh and warm.

Nutritional Values: Calories: 127; Total Fat: 4 g; Carbohydrates: 14 g; Protein: 9 g; Fiber: 0.2 g; Potassium: 148 mg; Phosphorus: 89 mg; Sodium: 129 mg; Cholesterol: 21mg; Iron 1mg; Vitamin A: 25.8mcg; Vitamin C: 1mg

39. Spicy Cornbread

Preparation time: 10 minutes

Cooking time: 30 minutes

Servings: 8

Ingredients:

- 1 cup all-purpose white flour
- 1 cup plain cornmeal
- 1 tbsp sugar
- 2 tsp baking powder
- 1 tsp chili powder
- ¼ tsp black pepper

- 1 cup rice milk, unenriched or almond milk
- 1 egg
- 1 egg white
- 2 tbsp canola oil
- ½ cup scallions, finely chopped
- ¼ cup carrots, finely grated
- 1 garlic clove, minced
- Cooking spray

Directions:

1. Preheat your oven to 400 F.
2. Mix the flour with baking powder, sugar, cornmeal, pepper, and chili powder in a mixing bowl. Stir in oil, milk, egg white, and egg.
3. Mix well until it's smooth, then stir in carrots, garlic, and scallions. Then, stir well, spread the batter in an 8-inch baking pan greased with cooking spray.
4. Bake for 30 minutes until golden brown. Slice and serve fresh.

Nutritional Values: Calories: 188; Total Fat: 5 g; Carbohydrates: 31 g; Protein: 5 g; Fiber: 2 g; Potassium: 100 mg; Phosphorus: 81 mg; Sodium: 155 mg; Cholesterol: 80.7mg; Iron 2.6mg; Vitamin A: 225mcg; Vitamin C: 3.6mg

40. Sweet and Spicy Tortilla Chips

Preparation time: 10 minutes

Cooking time: 8 minutes

Servings: 6

Ingredients:

- ¼ cup butter
- 1 tsp brown sugar
- ½ tsp ground chili powder
- ½ tsp garlic powder
- ½ tsp ground cumin
- ¼ tsp ground cayenne pepper
- 6 flour tortillas, 6-inch size
- Cooking spray

Directions:

1. Warm your oven to 425 F. Grease a baking sheet using a cooking spray. Add all spices, brown sugar, and melted butter to a small bowl. Mix well and set this mixture aside.
2. Slice the tortillas into 8 wedges and brush them with the sugar mixture. Spread them on the baking sheet and bake them for 8 minutes. Serve fresh.

Nutritional Values: Calories: 115; Total Fat: 7 g; Carbohydrates: 11 g; Protein: 2 g; Fiber: 0.6 g; Potassium: 42 mg; Phosphorus: 44 mg; Sodium: 156 mg; Cholesterol: 15mg; Iron .3mg; Vitamin A: 0mcg; Vitamin C: 0mg

41. Addictive Pretzels

Preparation time: 10 minutes

Cooking time: 1 hour

Servings: 6

Ingredients:

- 1 (32 oz.) bag of unsalted pretzels
- 1 cup canola oil
- 2 tbsp seasoning mix
- 3 tsp garlic powder
- 3 tsp dried dill weed

Directions:

1. Preheat the oven to 175 F. Break the pretzels into pieces and place them on a baking pan.
2. Combine garlic powder and dill in a bowl; set aside half of the mixture.
3. Combine the remaining half with the seasoning mix and ¾ cup of canola oil in a mixing bowl. Brush a generous amount of this oil over the pretzels.
4. Bake for 1 hour, rotate the pieces, and bake for another 15 minutes.
5. Allow to cool before sprinkling with the remaining dill mixture and drizzled with additional oil. Serve hot and fresh.

Nutritional Values: Calories: 184; Total Fat: 8 g; Carbohydrates: 22 g; Protein: 2 g; Fiber: 1.0 g; Potassium: 43 mg; Phosphorus: 28 mg; Sodium: 60 mg; Cholesterol: 0mg; Iron 0.4mg; Vitamin A: 10.2mcg; Vitamin C: 0.6mg

42. Citrus Sesame Cookies

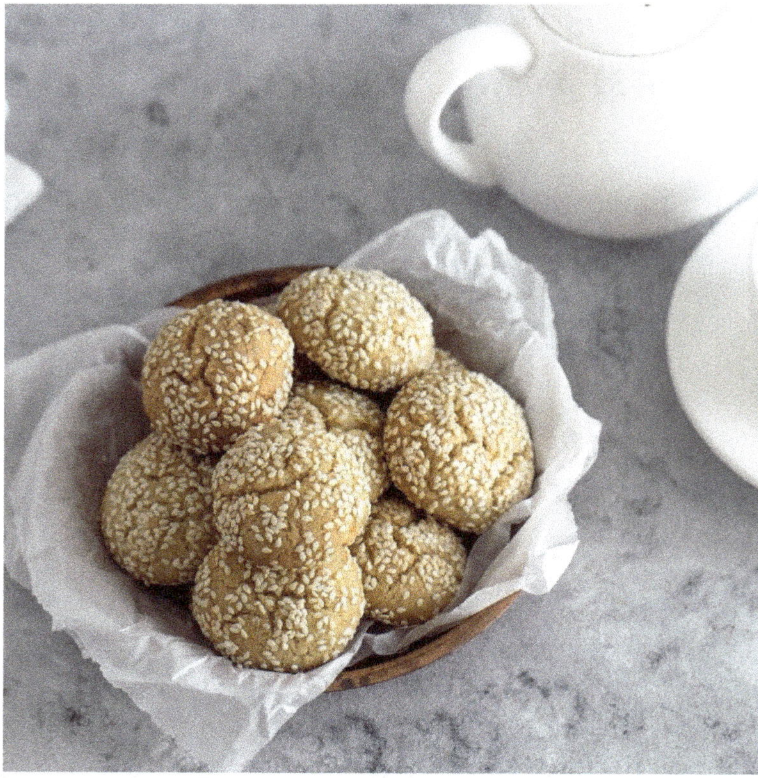

Preparation Time: 15 minutes + chilling time

Cooking time: 10 minutes

Servings: 18 cookies

Ingredients:

- ¾ cup unsalted butter, at room temperature

- ½ cup sugar
- 1 egg
- 1 teaspoon vanilla extract
- 2 cups all-purpose flour
- 2 tablespoons toasted sesame seeds
- ½ teaspoon baking soda
- 1 teaspoon freshly grated lemon zest
- 1 teaspoon freshly grated orange zest

Directions:

1. In your large bowl and using a mixer, beat together the butter and sugar on high speed until thick and fluffy, about 3 minutes.
2. Add the egg plus vanilla and beat to mix thoroughly, scraping down the sides of the bowl.
3. Stir together the flour, sesame seeds, baking soda, lemon zest, and orange zest in a small bowl.
4. Mix the flour mixture plus butter mixture, and stir until well blended.

5. Roll the dough into a long log-like about 2 inches diameter, and wrap in plastic wrap. Refrigerate for 1 hour.
6. Warm your oven to 350 F. Line a baking sheet using parchment paper. Cut the firm cookie dough into ½-inch-thick rounds, and place them on the prepared baking sheet.
7. Bake within 10 to 12 minutes until lightly golden. Cool completely on wire racks. Store in a sealed container in the refrigerator for up to 1 week or in the freezer for 2 months.

Nutritional Values: Calories: 150; Total Fat: 9g; Carbohydrates: 16g; Protein: 2g; Fiber: 1g; Phosphorus: 29mg; Potassium: 25mg; Sodium: 5mg; Cholesterol: 32mg; Iron 1.4mg; Vitamin A: 45mcg; Vitamin C: 0.3mg

43. Shrimp Spread with Crackers

Preparation time: 10 minutes

Cooking time: 0 minutes

Servings: 6

Ingredients:

- ¼ cup light cream cheese
- 2 ½ oz. cooked, shelled shrimp, minced
- 1 tbsp no-salt-added ketchup
- ¼ tsp hot sauce
- 1 tsp Worcestershire sauce
- ½ tsp herb seasoning blend
- 24 matzo cracker miniatures
- 1 tbsp parsley, minced

Directions:

1. Start by tossing the minced shrimp with cream cheese in a bowl. Stir in Worcestershire sauce, hot sauce, herb seasoning, and ketchup.
2. Mix well and garnish with minced parsley. Serve the spread with the crackers.

Nutritional Values: Calories: 57; Total Fat: 1 g, Carbohydrates: 7 g; Protein: 3 g; Fiber: 0.2 g; Potassium: 54 mg; Phosphorus: 30 mg; Sodium: 69 mg; Cholesterol: 20mg; Iron 0.2mg; Vitamin A: 85.5mcg; Vitamin C: 0.7mg

44. Chicken Pepper Bacon Wraps

Preparation time: 10 minutes

Cooking time: 15 minutes

Servings: 4

Ingredients:

- 2 lbs. boneless, skinless chicken breast
- 12 strips bacon, halved
- 12 fresh jalapenos peppers
- 12 fresh banana peppers
- 1 medium onion, chopped
- Cooking spray

Directions:

1. Grease a grill rack with cooking spray and preheat the grill on low heat. Slice

the peppers in half lengthwise, then remove their seeds.

2. Dice the chicken into small pieces and divide them into each pepper. Now spread the chopped onion over the chicken in the peppers.
3. Wrap the bacon strips around the stuffed peppers. Place these wrapped peppers in the grill and cook them for 15 minutes. Serve fresh and warm.

Nutritional Values: Calories: 71; Total Fat: 3 g; Carbohydrates: 1 g; Protein: 10 g; Fiber: 0.8 g; Potassium: 147 mg; Phosphorus: 84 mg; Sodium: 96 mg; Cholesterol: 17.6mg; Iron 0.4mg; Vitamin A: 55.9mcg; Vitamin C: 9.1mg

45. Garlic Oyster Crackers

Preparation time: 10 minutes

Cooking time: 45 minutes

Servings: 4

Ingredients:

- ½ cup butter-flavored popcorn oil
- 1 tbsp garlic powder
- 7 cups oyster crackers
- 2 tsp dried dill weed

Directions:

1. Preheat oven to 250 F. Mix garlic powder with oil in a large bowl. Toss in crackers and mix well to coat evenly.
2. Sprinkle the dill weed over the crackers and toss well again. Spread the crackers on the baking sheet and bake them for 45 minutes. Toss them every 15 minutes. Serve fresh.

Nutritional Values: Calories: 118; Total Fat: 7 g; Carbohydrates: 12 g; Protein: 2 g; Fiber: 3 g; Potassium: 21 mg; Phosphorus: 15 mg; Sodium: 166 mg; Cholesterol: 0mg; Iron 0.06mg; Vitamin A: 0mcg; Vitamin C: 0mg

46. Toasted Pear Chips

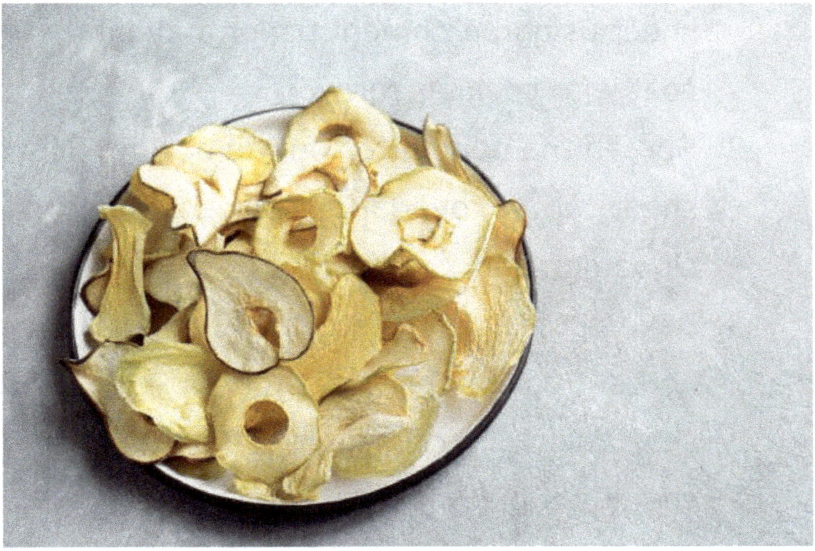

Preparation Time: 15 minutes

Cooking time: 3-4 hours

Servings: 4

Ingredients:

- 4 firm pears, cored and cut into 1/8-inch-thick slices
- 2 teaspoons ground cinnamon
- 1 tablespoon sugar
- Olive oil cooking spray

Directions:

1. Warm your oven to 200 F. Line a baking sheet using parchment paper and lightly coat with cooking spray.
2. Spread the pear slices on the baking sheet with no overlap. Sprinkle with cinnamon and sugar.
3. Bake until the chips are dry, 3 to 4 hours. Cool completely. Store in your sealed container for up to 4 days in a cool, dark place.

Nutritional Values: Calories: 101; Total Fat: 0g; Carbohydrates: 27g; Protein: 1g Fiber: 5g; Phosphorus: 17mg; Potassium: 183mg; Sodium: 2mg; Cholesterol: 0mg; Iron 0mg; Vitamin A: 0mcg; Vitamin C: 3mg

47. Sugar & Spice Popcorn

Preparation Time: 10 minutes

Cooking Time: 10 minutes

Servings: 4-5

Ingredients:

- 8 cups hot popcorn
- 2 tablespoons unsalted butter
- 2 tablespoons sugar
- 1/2 teaspoon cinnamon
- 1/4 teaspoon nutmeg

Directions:

1. Heat the butter, sugar, cinnamon, and nutmeg in the microwave or saucepan over a range fire until the butter is melted and the sugar is dissolved.
2. Sprinkle the popcorn with the spicy butter, mix well. Serve immediately for optimal flavor.

Nutritional Values: Calories: 120; Total Fat: 7g; Carbohydrates: 12g; Protein: 2g; Fiber 0g; Potassium: 56mg; Phosphorus: 60mg; Sodium: 2mg; Cholesterol: 0.1mg; Iron 0.1mg; Vitamin A: 31.05mcg; Vitamin C: 0mg

48. Baked Pita Fries

Preparation Time: 5 minutes

Cooking Time: 15 minutes

Servings: 6

Ingredients:

- 3 pita loaves (6 inches)
- 3 tablespoons olive oil
- Chili powder, as you like

Directions:

1. Separate each bread in half with scissors to obtain 6 round pieces. Cut each piece into eight points. Brush each using olive oil and sprinkle with chili powder.
2. Bake at 350 F for about 15 minutes until crisp. Serve and enjoy!

Nutritional Values: Calories: 120; Total Fat: 2.5g; Carbohydrates: 22g; Protein: 3g; Fiber 3g; Potassium: 0mg; Phosphorus: 0mg;

Sodium: 70mg; Cholesterol: 0mg; Iron 0.75mg; Vitamin A: 0mcg; Vitamin C: 0mg

49. Herbal Cream Cheese Tartines

Preparation Time: 15 minutes

Cooking Time: 15 minutes

Servings: 2

Ingredients:

- 1 clove garlic, halved
- 1 cup cream cheese spread
- ¼ cup chopped herbs such as chives, dill, parsley, tarragon, or thyme
- 2 tbsp. minced French shallot or onion
- ½ tsp. black pepper
- 2 tbsp. tablespoons water

Directions:

1. Combine the cream cheese, herbs, shallot, pepper, and water in a medium-sized bowl with a hand blender.
2. Serve the cream cheese with the rusks.

Nutritional Values: Calories: 476; Total Fat: 9g; Carbohydrates: 75g; Protein: 23g; Fiber 1g; Potassium: 312mg; Phosphorus: 165mg; Sodium: 885mg; Cholesterol: 51.89mg; Iron 0.7mg; Vitamin A: 0mcg; Vitamin C: 7.3mg

50. Eggplant and Chickpea Bites

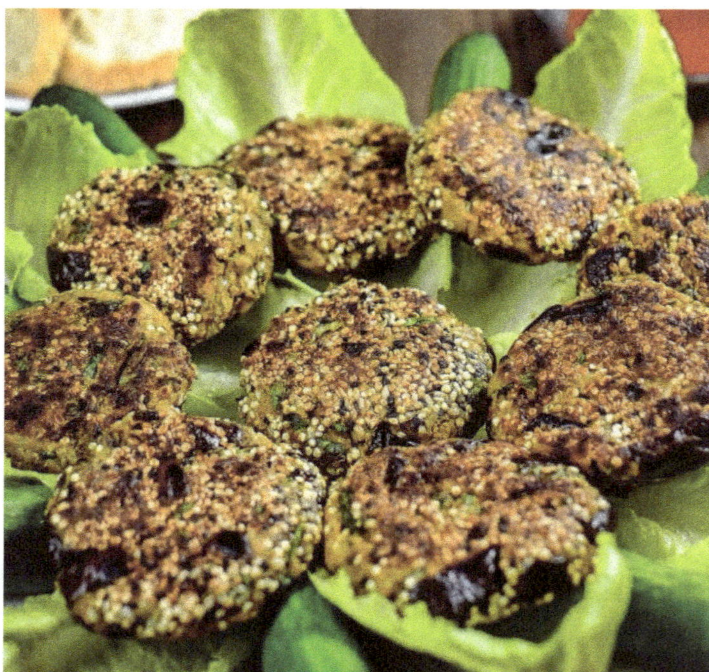

Preparation Time: 15 minutes

Cooking Time: 50 minutes

Servings: 6

Ingredients:

- 3 large eggplants cut in half (make a few cuts in the flesh with a knife)
- 2 large cloves garlic, peeled and deglazed
- 2 tbsp. coriander powder
- 2 tbsp. cumin seeds
- 2 cups canned chickpeas, rinsed and drained
- 2 tbsp chickpea flour
- Zest and juice of 1/2 lemon
- 1/2 lemon quartered for serving
- 3 tbsp. tablespoon of polenta

Directions:

1. Heat the oven to 392 F. Spray the eggplant halves generously with oil and place them on the meat side up on a baking sheet.
2. Sprinkle with coriander and cumin seeds, and then place garlic cloves on the plate.

3. Season and roast for 40 minutes until the flesh of the eggplant is completely tender. Reserve and let cool a little.
4. Scrape the flesh of the eggplant in a bowl with a spatula and throw the skins in the compost. Thoroughly scrape and make sure to incorporate spices and crushed roasted garlic.
5. Add chickpeas, chickpea flour, zest, and lemon juice. Crush roughly and mix well.
6. Check to season. Do not worry if the mixture seems a bit soft - it will firm up in the fridge.
7. Form about twenty pellets and place them on a baking sheet covered with parchment paper. Refrigerate for at least 30 minutes.
8. Preheat oven to 356 F. Remove the meatballs from the fridge and coat them by rolling them in the polenta.

9. Place them back on the baking sheet and spray a little oil on each. Roast for 20 minutes until golden and crisp.
10. Serve with lemon wedges. You can also serve these dumplings with a spicy yogurt dip.

Nutritional Values: Calories: 72; Total Fat: 1g; Carbohydrates: 18g; Protein: 3g; Fiber 2g; Potassium: 162mg; Phosphorus: 36mg; Sodium: 63mg; Cholesterol: 16mg; Iron 1mg; Vitamin A: 45.3mcg; Vitamin C: 3mg

28-DAY MEAL PLAN

DAY	BREAKFAST SMOOTHIE	LUNCH	DINNER	SNACKS
1	Vanilla Chia Smoothie	Aromatic Chicken and Cabbage Stir-Fry	Roasted Cod with Plums	Cinnamon Apple Chips
2	Mango Cheesecake Smoothie	Vegetable Beef Stir-Fry	Crustless Cabbage Quiche	Eggplant and Chickpea Bites
3	Raspberry Cucumber Smoothie	Chicken with Apricots	Mediterranean Eggplant Casserole	Roasted Onion Dip (with your favorite vegetabl

				e sticks or low-sodium crackers)
4	Melon Smoothie	Corn and Shrimp Quiche	Chicken, Pasta, and Broccoli Bake	Baked Pita Fries
5	Blackberry Kale Smoothie	Creamy Mushroom Pasta	Pineapple-Soy Salmon Stir-Fry	Sugar & Spice Popcorn
6	Apple Pie Smoothie	Oven-Fried Fish with Pineapple Salsa	Meatloaf with Mushroom Gravy	Toasted Pear Chips

7	Chocolate Smoothie	Ratatouille-Inspired Skewers	White Fish and Broccoli Curry	Garlic Oyster Crackers
8	Green Coconut Smoothie	Creamy Pesto Pasta	Pepper Jack and Rice Stuffed Peppers	Chicken Pepper Bacon Wraps
9	Creamy Dandelion Greens and Celery Smoothie	Roasted Veggie Sandwiches	Ginger Shrimp with Snow Peas	Shrimp Spread with Crackers
10	Almonds with Zucchini Smoothie	Chicken Patties with Dill	White Bean Veggie Burgers	Baba Ghanoush Dip (with your favorite

				vegetable sticks or low-sodium crackers)
11	Acai Berry Smoothie Bowl	Pork Tenderloin with Roasted Fruit	Mediterranean Cod	Citrus Sesame Cookies
12	Green Power Smoothie	Lemon Garlic Halibut	Baked Herbed Chicken	Addictive Pretzels
13	Watermelon Cucumber Smoothie	Spicy Corn and Rice Burritos	Red Pepper Pasta	Sweet and Spicy Tortilla Chips

14	Peach-Pineapple Protein Smoothie	Roasted Salmon with Herb Gremolata	Spinach Alfredo Lasagna Rolls	Spicy Cornbread
15	Berry Beet Smoothie Bowl	Tofu and Rice Salad Bowl	Turkey and Corn Chowder	Sweet Savory Meatballs
16	Mango Lassi Smoothie	Chicken Chow Mein	Cauliflower and Potato Curry	Cucumbers with Sour Cream (with your favorite vegetable sticks or low-sodium

				crackers)
17	Strawberry Spice Smoothie	Spicy Tofu and Broccoli Stir-Fry	Chicken Breast and Bok Choy in Parchment	Roasted Garlic White Bean Dip (with your favorite vegetable sticks or low-sodium crackers)
18	Peach Melba Smoothie	Roasted Onion Clam Chowder	Rice-Stuffed Mini Meatloaves	Spicy Buffalo Cauliflower Bites

19	Blueberry Burst Smoothie	Red Beans and Rice	Turkey Meatballs and Spaghetti in Garlic Sauce	Honey-Vanilla Energy Balls
20	Cucumber Spinach Green Smoothie	Marinated Pork Tenderloin	Salmon and Kale in Parchment	Herbal Cream Cheese Tartines
21	Strawberry Cheesecake Smoothie	Cabbage-Stuffed Mushrooms	Lemon-Butter Tilapia	Roasted Red Pepper Hummus (with your favorite vegetable sticks or low-sodium

				crackers)
22	Raspberry Peach Smoothie	Shrimp Skewers with Mango Cucumber Salsa	Flank Steak with Chimichurri Sauce	Savory Collard Chips
23	Watermelon Kiwi Smoothie	Spinach Falafel Wrap	Lemon Chicken	Parmesan Roasted Cauliflower
24	Strawberry, Raspberry, & Kale Smoothie	Ginger-Orange Tuna Pasta Salad	Peanut-Chili Tofu with Noodles	Baked Jicama Fries

25	Blueberry, Strawberry, & Cauliflower Smoothie	Chicken Satay with Peanut Sauce	Creamy Veggie Casserole	Fruit Dip (with your favorite fruits or low-sodium crackers)
26	Vanilla Chia Smoothie	Vegetable Beef Stir-Fry	Chicken, Pasta, and Broccoli Bake	Cinnamon Apple Chips
27	Mango Cheesecake Smoothie	Chicken with Apricots	Mediterranean Cod	Eggplant and Chickpea Bites

28	Melon Smoothie	Corn and Shrimp Quiche	Crustless Cabbage Quiche	Roasted Onion Dip (with your favorite vegetable sticks or low-sodium crackers)

CPSIA information can be obtained
at www.ICGtesting.com
Printed in the USA
LVHW081647040322
712645LV00006B/517

9 781803 034836